The Marathon Scam

Why You Should Never Run a Marathon and If You Do,
How to Avoid Serious Injury

by Ed SJC Park

First Edition: 2012

ISBN 978-1-300-51457-2

Acknowledgments

Phil S., Eric L., Josh, Laura F., Ingrid, and Skechers

Contents

Introduction

Imagine millions of people deciding to become bodybuilders and within a 20-week training period attempt to bench 400 pounds, or ride a bull, race a Formula One car at 200 MPH, parachute from 30,000 feet solo, fly an airplane solo into a storm, ride a bicycle 2,000 miles in a month like in the Tour de France, climb Mt. Everest, surf 100-foot waves, or eat 50 hot dogs in ten minutes. Undoubtedly, you would have millions of people sustain serious injuries, perhaps become crippled for life or die. Yet, millions of people try to run marathons not only because it is so inexpensive and accessible, but also because of the hype.

It is irresponsible for marathon guides and blogs to encourage the public to train for a marathon in 20-weeks or even run one. Most people simply do not have the patience or time to properly train for a marathon which I believe takes at least a year. Their excess weight also contributes to injuries along with shoes designed to injure them. It takes at least a year to transition into proper minimalist running shoes without any type of theatrical, unscientific support system. It takes at least a year for your body to naturally heal and build up for a 26.2 mile super endurance endeavor. The vast majority of injuries are a result of inadequate rest and recovery time. Given a strict 20-week regiment, people push themselves through injury aggravating it and during the marathon itself, push themselves well beyond the pain threshold causing in many cases permanent injury. Support shoes not only contribute to injuries by misinforming the body about the surface tension and hardness, but they mask pain, allowing you to run further on injury and create worse problems in the long-run.

The sheer number of both minor and major injuries in marathon training should be a warning sign to everyone, yet marathon enthusiasts keep raving about marathons for everyone. If as many people sustained all these injuries from walking up a certain flight of stairs, wouldn't you think those stairs are dangerous? Wouldn't you fix those stairs and quit blaming the people getting injured? The majority of people training for a marathon sustain injuries. If the majority of people driving cars had accidents, isn't it about time to quit blaming driver error and start redesigning cars, roads, and traffic signals?

For the average person, training for and running in a marathon is not healthy. If you want to become a fit, well-conditioned athlete, there are many other ways to do this with substantially less injury including running a 20k or half-marathon. This is like trying to develop a properly balanced, healthy diet by becoming a competitive eater. You are pushing yourself beyond normal, natural boundaries thinking the more you push yourself, the healthier you will become when in fact you simply increase the chance for injury and/or wind up hating the activity for life. Surely, many people run marathons injury-free and are very healthy, and Takeru Kobayashi, a world champion competitive eater is the model of fitness, however, the majority of us would get sick from competitive eating and probably damage our esophagus from throwing up so much food. Why risk your health for a pointless, random distance?

However, should you fall prey to your inflated and fragile ego and get suckered into the marathon scam; my advice is not limited to abstinence. This book will provide you with safe tips for training that will reduce your chances of injury in your pointless, reckless, irrational pursuit of marathon glory. Having been injured and completed a marathon in 2012, I have fresh advice in mind in a concise format that may complement a more comprehensive marathon training book or substitute it for light readers.

About the Author

I am not one of those obese, sedentary fast-food junkies who decided to lose weight by running a marathon. I have kept fit all my life and never been overweight. In high school, I joined a bicycle racing club. I won a few junior state championships and made it to Junior Olympic Training Camp. I read U.S. National Coaching Director, Eddie Borysewicz's famous book, *Bicycle Road Racing: The Complete Program for Training and Competition.* I studied training to get the maximum possible advantage possible. I wasn't the best, and I realized in bicycle racing, unless you are the best, you don't really have much of a future in it. Of course, today, whether a sprinter or endurance bicycle racer, you really can't win unless you're doping your brains out.

After high school, I focused on weight lifting and then started running to help friends get in shape. One day, for whatever crazed reason, I tried to beat my all-time distance record of 8 miles. I was about to turn 42. Maybe it was a mid-life crisis thing. I hit 10 miles, but I had never experienced so much pain in my life, at least not that I could recall. My right knee finally gave out, and I hobbled the last mile. It was excruciating. So why then did I then entertain the possibility of running a marathon? Stupidity and vanity. Actually, the endorphins that are released into your system, your body's natural painkillers, are probably the reason why so many people get addicted to long-distance running.

Like most people, I imagine, I thought I could wing it. I would browse the Internet for marathon advice, but for the most part wing it, solo. I got a 20-week, novice training schedule online. I talked to a friend who had run a marathon. I thought I was good to go. Then I got injured.

After getting injured, I finally took it seriously and hit the books in exasperation. I bought a stupid eBook that was a waste of $5 when I should have just bought *Runner's World Big Book of Marathon and Half-Marathon Training*. Curious about the whole minimalist shoe trend, I also bought *Tread Lightly: Form, Footwear, and the Quest for Injury-Free Running*. While all the information I received in these books and online was immensely helpful, I realized that training for and running a marathon are unhealthy endeavors, especially with only 20-weeks to train. I realized I had the wrong shoes. I realized I didn't give myself enough time to adapt to better shoes. I realized that after having paid the registration fee and airplane tickets for the marathon, I had placed myself on an irreversible course of self-destruction, tempting fate, recklessness, aggravating my injuries, and risking permanent disability. Despite better common sense, I pushed forward like an addict in denial, but I hope my book will help others avoid the delusional ego-pit I fell into or at least prepare better to avoid injury.

Pre-Decision

Why Modern Humans Should NOT Be Running Marathons

In 490 BC, some Greek messenger was dispatched from the city of Marathon to Athens to announce that the Greeks had defeated the Persians at the Battle of Marathon. Then he died. Now, you wonder, why the hell does everyone want to go run a distance that is so long the first dude whoever did it died? And how arbitrary is that distance? What if the cities were five miles apart or fifty? Would everyone be running 5-mile marathons or going for 50-mile marathons? 26.2 is like 2.998×10^8 m/sec, the speed of light. There's no reason why it's 2.998×10^8 it just is. Why is one route between Marathon and Athens 26.2 miles? The Anthropic Principle would argue that the only reason it's 26.2 miles is that if it were not 26.2 miles, we would not exist in a world where we would be able to ask that question. Personally, I think it's just stupid randomness.

26.2 miles is not natural and in fact a dangerous distance to cover all in one go, over the same terrain. Even worse, course time limits are forcing people to push themselves toward permanent injury. Ancient humans may have covered 26.2 miles over the course of a day, but they often walked and stopped for breaks. While the human is specially designed to run long distances, especially in the heat, they are not designed to run continually on the same surface for 26.2 miles. When hunting animals, the terrain changes constantly, and hunters alternated between jogging, walking, stopping, sprinting, jogging, and walking. The marathon is a boon to the medical/healthcare industry. Even those who finish a marathon, even the ones who are not crippled, often quit running altogether from the trauma. The marathon is an unnatural, purely ego-driven exercise in self-destruction. Personal enlightenment and spiritual growth? Please. Hitting yourself in the forehead 40,000 times and gradually developing the thick skull and persistence to do it all in one go without knocking yourself unconscious will give you the same personal enlightenment and spiritual growth as running a marathon.

Humans are also designed for strength and power. Why else would we have fast-twitch bulk muscle in addition to slow-twitch endurance muscles? Humans are truly one of the most flexible animals around. We can also eat a mostly meat or vegetarian diet. Just because we can run long distances does not mean we should.

The average modern human is also in no way designed to run a marathon. The average American is overweight. All that weight multiplies the pressure placed on all your joints and ligaments. I highly doubt ancient humans were overweight and running 26.2 miles. Unless, you are retired or living on a trust fund, the average American also does not have the time to not only properly train for a marathon but properly recover from workouts. At work, the stress, all day sitting, and energy expended at work significantly diminish our body's ability to recovery and develop in 20 weeks for a 26.2-mile effort. On top of this, let us not forget the countless toxins modern humans suffer including life-long cumulative exposure to air pollution, smoking, alcohol, cholesterol, fat, salt, toxic unnatural ingredients, hormones, antibiotics, preservatives, etc. Sure you pick up a 100,000 year-old human in a time machine, train him for 20 weeks, and he would do very well with minimal injury, but let me know when you get that time machine working.

The average person also has grown up with the wrong shoes. I will get into this more under Pre-Training. Recently, we have created factory food that is killing us, but we have also created factory shoes that are injuring us. Today's shoes are way too constrictive, suffocating, rigid, and padded. As a result, our feet are too small, infected with fungus, have bunions, and all our joints suffer. While you may blame cars for making us sedentary and unfit, you can also blame our factory shoes for making walking and running painful. The Chinese used to bind women's feet to make them small. Today's factory shoes are a similar form of binding for aesthetic purposes with dramatically negative health side-effects. Unfortunately, on these deformed feet, the average person is ill-suited to run 26.2 miles and it takes at least a year for us to adapt to proper shoes, although, arguably, our bodies will never fully adapt to proper shoes after a lifetime of foot-binding.

Marathons Are For Nerds

I never wanted to do long-distance running, because I never wanted to look like a long-distance runner. Elite marathon runners look anorexic with chicken legs. I find this about as natural as a body builder on steroids with veins popping out larger than my muscles. As mentioned above, the human is designed for either strength or endurance or both. This flexibility has allowed humans to adapt to all sorts of different situations. Some humans had to chase animals for 30 miles to get a meal while others sprinted a hundred yards or built up muscle mass to fight off other humans. While I applaud long-distance runners for their athleticism, I also applaud sprinters and boxers for their athleticism, but as a guy, I applaud MMA fighters the most for their strength and fighting skills. As far as I'm concerned, I'd rather look like an MMA fighter and having their fighting skills too. We don't live in a world where we have to chase an animal down 30 miles for food or physically fight another dude for a woman, but it is more likely that we will need to use our fighting strength and skill more than our long-distance running abilities.

Probably for this reason, there are now more female runners than male runners. Many women use running as a way to not only keep in shape but to keep the weight off in a society that has become obsessed with slim, almost anorexic female bodies. Even then, I believe that training for and running a half-marathon is a hundred times more healthy and beneficial than trying to run a full marathon.

20K is the Better Way

If your goal in life is to become fit and enjoy long-distance running, the ideal distance is 20K or what is referred to as a "half-marathon." It is unfortunate that it is called a "half-marathon" which makes you think it is "half-ass" or "half-way." Would you go on a half-vacation, drive a half-car, eat a half-steak, marry a half-man, watch a half-weight fight? Running a 20K will give you the same rewards and personal growth minus the injury. Running a 20K for the average American is a noble, worthwhile goal, and not only are you significantly less likely to get injured, but you are significantly more likely to enjoy it and spend the rest of your life running 20K and loving and enjoying running injury free. Even expert marathon runners get serious injuries running 26.2 miles. A marathon is not truly an endurance sport but rather an injury evasion sport like running with the bulls or freestyle climbing without ropes. You don't do it for the endurance aspect but the thrill of not getting seriously injured.

Even better, the terrain and speed should constantly be varied. They should then detour the route into parks and even have hurdles. The modern marathon is a disaster and almost seems like the perfect storm to maximize injuries and suffering. In this sense, it is about as unhealthy as competitive eating. Certainly, you can train yourself to be an excellent competitive eater but also at a heavy cost to your health. I very much doubt ancient humans ran so far they permanently injured themselves. It just doesn't make any sense. They most likely realized the hunt was not worth weeks, months, perhaps years of disability and cut their losses and quit. "Hey look, Huga is hobbling and does not stop running. Huga too proud. Huga will be out for months. Huga will starve. We will split Huga's possessions and bury him. Dibs on Huga's wife."

Why Training for a Marathon is an Awful Weight Loss Plan

If you want to lose weight, you need to gradually eat less and exercise more. Jumping into a marathon, your body will go into shock and learn to hate exercise, and your appetite will actually increase. The reason many people are overweight is because they eat junk food which delivers little nutrition at an exorbitant cost of calories. Training for a marathon, your body will crave even more nutrition, but if you're already so used to getting your nutrients through junk food, your body will simply go crazy craving massive quantities of junk food. Trust me on this, training for a marathon will give you an endless appetite for food.

Even worse, if you already carry excess weight, your chances of getting injured almost increase exponentially. Give an elite marathon runner a 50-pound backpack, and there is a good chance he'll start suffering joint pains and sprains. When you are injured and cannot exercise properly, you'll have this insatiable athlete's appetite and no exercise to burn it, so you'll gain even more weight. If you truly want goals to help you lose weight, give yourself a realistic, sustainable goal. Try to run a 10K or 20K every year of your life for the rest of your life. You are much more likely to 1. enjoy running and exercise, 2. avoid injury, and 3. lose weight. The marathon scam is perhaps most damaging to people who try to do it to lose weight. Running a marathon to lose weight is like screaming for five hours straight to become a better singer.

Minimizing Damage

However, if you are stupid and egotistical like me, you want to run a marathon, because it has bragging rights and sustaining a life-long injury and possibly being deterred from ever running long-distance again is worth the potential glory. I swear, if you ever watch the end of a marathon after 5 hours it looks like zombie land. Hobbling with pain cannot be good for you. These people are hurting themselves, possibly for life. So what if their will power is greater than their pain threshold. That is not inspiring; it's pure stupidity. Is it inspiring to watch a monkey spend all day trying to get an orange out of a jar when all he has to do is let go and roll the jar upside down? After finishing my stupid marathon, I truly want to run half-marathons the rest of my life and leave the marathon to people not only who have the time and talent for it, but people stupid enough to try it. Half-marathons are for the intelligent folk who have made enjoyable, injury-free running a lifestyle choice. Unless you have a nice trust fund and don't have to work, you can put in the hours to build up your body and minimize injury in a marathon, but seriously, join the Peace Corps and do something a little bit more meaningful with your life.

Don't take a marathon lightly. Don't think you can just wing it and use pure instinct and determination. If you take the marathon lightly and just wing it, A) you will likely not finish the marathon and B) you will likely sustain a serious injury that you may have to live with the rest of your life.

There is a lot of good marathon advice out there just like advice for going to Burning Man or traveling in general. Sure, you want to improvise and do your own thing, but you also want to be prepared so you have even greater freedom to improvise and do your own thing. Seek and take advice. This is not the time to rely solely on yourself. The main goal of a marathon should not be finishing it. **The main goal of a marathon is finishing it without sustaining life-long injuries.** This is like saying, I want to make a million dollars at all costs, and afterwards, you have lost all your friends and family, your soul, and sooner or later, the police will arrest you for fraud. You want to finish the marathon, but you don't want to spend the rest of your life regretting it with incessant joint pain, back soreness, and arthritis. It saddens me to hear of so many stories of people who tried to or ran a marathon and suffered life-long injuries.

Are you ready for pain, sacrifice, and commitment? Most people run a marathon for the bragging rights, and that's just fine, but finishing a marathon is not impressive because it means you're physically talented like a race horse. It means you have the tenacity, discipline, determination, and commitment to a plan as well as stupidity. People often confuse discipline. They think that if they are disciplined in general, they can do anything that requires discipline. Discipline is a misnomer. It really describes consistent motivation. Someone who is highly motivated to finish a marathon may not be consistently motivated (disciplined) enough to train properly. They can be "disciplined" at work and school, but they lack the consistent motivation for marathon training. Being disciplined in one area does not translate into being disciplined in another. "Discipline" or rather consistent motivation is task dependent. A Navy SEAL may be "disciplined" enough to pass BUDS, but make him babysit a spoiled brat and he may quit after a few minutes. You think some pothead may not be "disciplined" enough to finish school, but give him a guitar or something he finds enjoyable, and he may practice several hours a day, seven days a week. The only reason people are not "disciplined" or consistently motivated for a specific task is because 1. the task itself is not immediately rewarding, 2. there is no one providing social reinforcement, and 3. the end goal is not clearly defined or provides no rewards. Anyone can get over any discomfort or pain if these three criteria are met.

Pre-Training

Shoes

The three most important equipment for runners: shoes, shoes, and shoes

Besides going out too fast, too soon, the largest cause of injuries is footwear. Before you even take your first step outside training, make sure you have the right shoes to cover 26.2 miles injury free. Finishing a marathon is a great accomplishment, but when you do it all costs and get a lifelong injury, you won't be looking back at the marathon as the pinnacle of your physical accomplishments. You'll be looking back at the marathon as the start of lifelong pain and misery. I cannot emphasis more how much you do not want to injury yourself during training, and shoes and your training schedule will dictate whether you finish the marathon injury free or injured for life.

The Skinny on Minimalist Shoes

There is a raging debate these days over minimalist and support shoe running. There is less debate over barefoot running, because that's just crazy and in an urban environment, you really don't want to be running over broken glass and nails and have to get tetanus shots. Here are some basic arguments from both sides:

Support shoes: While humans have evolved without support shoes, we have also evolved without hard roads. Perhaps minimalist shoes work for trail running, but on hard road surfaces (most marathons are run on the road), it is essential to have some support and cushioning. Most of us also grew up with shoes, and over a lifetime have adapted to walking and running in shoes. When you switch to minimalist shoes, your body must readapt decades of muscle memory and habit. Without arch support for those who over-pronate, they are more likely to sustain injuries. It takes a long time to train the body to avoid over-pronating, and even longer the heavier you are. Minimalist shoes work for people who already have perfect running form and can adapt quickly.

Over-pronation happens when you hit the ground first with the outside of your heel then roll across diagonally to the inside of your midsole and off the inside ball of your foot. All the while, your toes are pointed to the side, so you look like a duck. It puts tremendous pressure on your inside ankle ligaments.

Minimalist shoes: When you run with support shoes, it puts all your body out-of-line and as a result, you will suffer back, hip, knee, shin, and ankle pain and injuries. Humans evolved over about 200K years without shoes. In the winter time, they may have covered their feet with animal skins, but there was no padding, arch support, etc. Humans are natural long-distance runners, and only during modern times with the introduction of support shoes have humans begun to suffer countless joint injuries all related to their shoes. Support shoes buffer the essential feedback from the ground your entire body needs to adjust itself. Imagine lifting weights with boxing gloves. You won't be able to feel the subtle movement of the weight as you lift so you may tend to overstrain one muscle instead of compensating. Support shoes also hide and abet poor running form, running with your feet splayed instead of straight, heel striking instead of mid-sole striking, etc. Support shoes may build up your leg muscles, but their cushioning properties leave your ligaments and tendons weak, the very mechanisms that put a spring in your step and reduce joint stress. As a result, over time, you not only suffer joint damage but eventually you suffer ligament and tendon strains and sprains.

Here's my personal story: Before training for a marathon, I depended on my decade+ old Skechers cross-trainers that were not flexible and had a huge heel. I never had problems with them until I started doing distance running (10+ miles) and learned that the big heel causes tremendous stress on my knee joints and back. As a result, my right knee had acute pain and I suffered horrible back spasms and a constant sore and stiff back. With 7.5 weeks to go to the marathon, knowing that you're not supposed to switch horses mid-stream, I decided to buy Skechers GoRun's, a transition into minimalist shoes with stiffer cushioning in the midsole and a small heel to encourage mid-foot striking. (It is the same with professional wrestling falls. They spread their bodies so they fall on their back, arms, and feet to distribute the impact force.) They appeared to be a lifesaver and both my knee and back pain disappeared. It is also quite possible that my knee and back simply became stronger.

(Disclaimer: I am in no way, shape, or form getting anything from Skechers. This is not one of those evil, guerilla marketing ploys to sell product. I've just simply always liked Skechers style, and fact is their performance running shoes, especially the minimalist ones, are some of the best and cheapest on the market.)

Then I did my 20-miler and the week after doing speed intervals, my hip started to hurt and I had a minor right interior ankle sprain. Thinking my problem was over-pronation, I looked for a shoe with interior foot support for over-pronators. (The real problem was that I had given myself long enough time to transition into these semi-minimalist shoes, and my ligaments and tendons were still weak.) I came across the Brooks Addiction line which seemed to be optimal for over-pronators with almost orthopedic looking interior midsole support and a wide midsole. I settled on the Brooks Infiniti 2 with moderate over-pronation support. I went out for a 4-mile run and low-and-behold, my knee and back pain returned as I must have started to heel-strike again with all that cushioning on the heel. I went back to my GoRun's but I could definitely feel my ankle again, so I tried out the Brooks Adrenaline GTS 11, and I could barely notice my ankle although my back became a little stiff again. I ran the last two weeks on the GoRun's with additional arch support insoles, but I then ran the entire marathon with the Brooks Adrenaline GTS 11. At Mile 23 I cramped, however, and hobbled/jogged the rest of the way.

I'll try minimalist again, but it will much more gradual. What I learned is that not only do support shoes rob you of the feel for the ground, but they also mask pain. I can certainly run in my Brooks support shoes and not feel my sore ankle as much, but fact is, I really shouldn't be running a lot on my bad ankle. By masking pain, support shoes lead to more serious injuries. It's like the old paradigm of fighting every small forest fire which leads to the buildup of forest floor debris which in turn leads to even larger forest fires. By running so close to the ground, you also feel your body pains more, and you run less until your body has properly recovered. A lot of boxers suffer wrist injuries from the constant pounding of their fists into punching bags. Their padded gloves allow them to punch significantly harder, yet imagine if they did not have heavily padded gloves. They would not hit as hard feeling the pain, but perhaps over time, their knuckles would harden and over this period, their wrist ligaments would also strengthen properly to sustain the punishment. Perhaps our bodies are a lot wiser than we give them credit.

Minimalist running may be better for you in the long run, but let us get one thing perfectly clear. If you have spent your entire life with shoes with a lot of cushioning and support, it will take a long, long time before your body will fully adjust to minimalist running. In other words, **you should ease into it with slow, easy runs not speed or endurance runs right before a marathon.** It is quite possible that it would take an entire year for your body to adapt to minimalist shoes and build up the necessary tendon and ligament strength to run an entire marathon without injury. Think of it this way. Some martial artists kick and punch without padding to harden up the bones on their fist, feet, and shins. However, with eight weeks before a tournament, after always wearing padding, do you want to switch to no-padding and arrive at the tournament with sore and swollen fists, feet, and shins that have actually reduced your training time?

Skecher GoRun's are somewhat controversial themselves. The midsole cushioning is stiffer and taller than the front or heel. It literally feels like you're running on a tiny bump in your shoe. For me, the invaluable benefit is that I never heel strike which has eliminated my knee and back pain. But minimalism is minimalism, and this means at some point, you have to go without the midsole hump and transition into a true minimalist shoe with consistently little cushioning throughout the entire sole.

Heels, WTF?

The minimalist debate is mostly about how much cushioning you have between the ground and your feet, but the most obvious problem everyone seems to ignore is not the amount of cushioning but the placement of that cushioning. Humans are designed to run on all types of terrain whether sand, mud, grass, hard-packed soil, or rock. It makes sense that you can put anything on the sole of shoes, and humans will adapt their running style to fit that artificial surface. However, WTF is with the heel? Where on Earth and even on Mars is there a surface out there where you will always land on a slightly raised surface on your heel?

Imagine walking barefoot across small cobblestones. Do you put your heel on the cobblestone and let your toes sink into the space between the cobblestones? This makes no sense whatsoever and sounds painful. Most sane people would tiptoe across the cobblestones or at least hit them midsole. Only the village idiot would walk around on his heels on cobblestones, and he would be the only one with major back problems. Whatever you think about the minimalist shoe debate, you have to agree that the raised heel is unnatural and forces people to constantly touch down on their heels. Just put on your shoes and try walking on the tip of your toes or midsole. Every time your heel strikes the ground first, the body is confused. It's expecting the midsole to strike first, but when the heel strikes, the body is not prepared and shock waves go up throughout the body.

The idea behind cushioned heels on running shoes is that they cushion your heel impact. However, this would only make sense if the heel compressed so much that it becomes level with the rest of the shoe sole. Have you ever seen this happen? Heels may be fine for standing around and being taller, but as far as running, heels should simply be banned. In fact, if you don't want to buy a new pair of running shoes without heels, simply get a saw and cut those heels off (of course, be extremely careful). If you go online for shoes, unfortunately, you are forced into two extremes: big heel support or bare minimal support all over. There are few shoes out there that have uniform support everywhere with no heel, what they call zero-drop. I think this would be the ideal shoe for the average person to start with. On top of this, evolutionarily speaking, humans have never had so much fat or for that matter muscle on their bodies. Perhaps modern humans do need some minimal, uniform cushioning.

Training Schedule

I believe most successful marathon runners are intelligent, disciplined nerds who know how to plan ahead, stick to a plan, and see a long-run goal through. That is their nature. They don't just jump into the deep end impulsively. Most unsuccessful marathon runners are either not intelligent and/or jock athletes unfamiliar with endurance sports who think they can just power through everything, push themselves to the limit until they reach 26.2 miles. The latter runners are unsuccessful, because they often get injured or demoralized and stop training. I like to compare marathon running to raising children. Studies show that the more structured and involved the parent is with children, the more successful the children. The parent has a plan and sticks to it consistently. Parents who just wing it are either too negligent or too controlling or alternate unpredictably between the two. They are impulsively reacting to their moods, the children's moods, or one problem after another. They either spoil the children and give in to their every discomfort and desire or they are too strict and completely ignore their every discomfort or desire. In training for a marathon, you need to be consistent and objectively attentive to your discomfort, pain, and enthusiasm. You should push yourself when you feel tired but never push yourself when you suffer consistent, acute pain. You should also learn to hold back and not over-train when you feel overly eager to do more mileage than planned or push yourself when injured. You should neither be lazy nor overly obsessive about your training schedule and push yourself too hard. You should be forgiving of your failures, consistent, patient, and trust yourself to come through in the end and succeed.

There are no if's, and's, or but's about it; you need a training schedule, and you need to keep at least 70% faithful to it. Now, here's advice that is probably worth the price of this book. Most all novice training schedules out there are too short at 20 weeks. They almost all will guarantee injury and excessive suffering during the marathon, perhaps permanent injury. Expert runners have simply forgotten the first time they started doing endurance runs. Perhaps it may have been as far back as high school. If you're a short-distance jock or someone who never ran more than two miles like me, you need more than 20 weeks to train for a marathon plain and simple.

The training schedule can be broken down into three different types of body conditioning. In the beginning, you're elevating your cardiovascular fitness, your ability to inhale oxygen and then pump that oxygen through your body. You're exercising your lungs and heart. You don't even need to run to do this, just any activity that elevates your breathing and heart rate. Interval training focuses on this by pushing your lungs and heart to the max. However, you don't want to do too much speed/interval training or else you'll develop fast-twitch, bulky muscles that will only slow you down for endurance work.

Once you have achieved an acceptable level of cardiovascular fitness and do not need to stop for air, the next step is building up your slow-twitch, endurance muscles. At this point, you can go on forever without losing your breath, but what stops you now is muscle fatigue. This is when you should be eating as much natural, organic protein as you can manage. Protein will also fix and strengthen your ligaments and tendons keeping you from injury. Most people do not realize that when you exercise, you are not only building and strengthening muscle fibers; you are also building and strengthening your ligaments, tendons, and even your bones. (The difference between a ligament and tendon is that ligaments connect bone to bone whereas tendons connect bone to muscles.) The more exercise and stress you place upon your ligaments, tendons, and bones, the stronger they become. Of course, you do not want to overstress them or else they will become sprained, strained, or broken. (A sprain only applies to ligaments whereas strains only apply to muscles and tendons.) This is one reason I feel padded shoes cause injuries. They do not allow us to place enough stress on our ligaments and tendons so that our muscles become stronger than the ligaments and tendons allowing us to run further but also making us exceedingly more vulnerable to ligament and tendon damage. Without padding, our ligaments and tendons are stressed and exercised allowing them to become stronger.

At this point, you should be doing your long runs at a very slow, steady, relaxed pace, never losing breath. If you start to hurt, simply slow down. You may feel that you're running too slow, but trust me, you need to build up your endurance muscles not your sprint muscles.

Finally, at about 14 miles, the final step is building up your energy efficiency. At 14 miles, it is not your muscles that give out but your entire body from energy depletion, right down to the cellular level. The only way to run 14 miles and more is to carb load the day before and then constantly take in quick carbs through easily digestible foods like bananas or carb gels. The only time you should ever use quick carbs is right before, during, and right after long runs. After 14 miles, you are training your body to process quick carbs to keep yourself from bonking.

Most training schedules are 20 weeks, but it really depends on how physically fit you are to begin with. You also have to decide whether you want to jog and walk the marathon or try to jog it all the way. I believe most training schedules for beginners are designed for you to jog and then walk the remaining four to six miles. If you want to jog the entire length anc stay injury free, I would suggest a longer training period. If you can't even jog two miles without getting sick or walking, then you should not start the one year program until you can. Then it's just a matter of finding a marathon in a year. My 48-week program allows you to miss a few target long runs. You don't want a 20-week plan where if you miss one long run the entire plan is messed up. I twice missed a target long run, first because of back pain and then because of a minor interior ankle sprain. It is simply unrealistic to stick precisely to a fixed plan for 20 weeks.

The typical training schedule will build you up to 10 miles in two-mile increments and then it will alternate between a long run and a recovery run with constant running or cross training throughout the week with one or two days of rest per week. With three weeks to go, it will give you a 20 mile run. They say 20 miles is sufficient, because every two weeks you're adding two miles, so for the marathon, they assume you'll be able to do 22 miles and then the last 4.2 miles you'll simply be feeding off all your adrenaline and the excitement of the crowds. I argue that the stress of running your first marathon, possibly in a new city, and all the crowds will sap your energy and you'll wind up walking the last 4.2 miles in agony. I would much rather jog the entire distance and end with manageable pain than tremendous suffering and agony and possible long-term injury. On top of that, I can't tell you how many people have told me how they seriously injured themselves training or running a marathon. I honestly think most 20-week training programs out there are unrealistic, irresponsible, and guarantee injury.

The 48-Week Injury Free Marathon Training Schedule

Part I – Cardio and Muscle Building

Week	Sun	Mon	Tue	Wed	Thu	Fri	Sat	Weekly

								Miles
1		Rest	1	Rest	Rest	1 EZ	Rest	2
2	2	Rest	1 EZ	Rest	Rest	1	Rest	4
3	2 int	Rest	CT	Rest	Rest	2 EZ	Rest	4
4	3	Rest	2 EZ	Rest	Rest	2	Rest	7
5	3 int	Rest	CT	Rest	Rest	2 EZ	Rest	5
6	4	Rest	2 EZ	Rest	Rest	2	Rest	8
7	3 int	Rest	CT	Rest	Rest	2 EZ	Rest	5
8	5	Rest	2 EZ	Rest	Rest	2	Rest	9
9	3 int	Rest	CT	Rest	Rest	2 EZ	Rest	5
10	6	Rest	2 EZ	Rest	Rest	4	Rest	12
11	4 int	Rest	CT	Rest	Rest	4 EZ	Rest	8
12	7	Rest	2 EZ	Rest	Rest	4	Rest	13
13	4 int	Rest	CT	Rest	Rest	4 EZ	Rest	8
14	8	Rest	2 EZ	Rest	Rest	4	Rest	14
15	4 int	Rest	CT	Rest	Rest	4 EZ	Rest	8
16	9	Rest	2 EZ	Rest	Rest	4	Rest	15
17	4 int	Rest	CT	Rest	Rest	4 EZ	Rest	8
18	10	Rest	2 EZ	Rest	Rest	4	Rest	16

CT=Cross Training/Cardio, int=intervals (not sprinting), EZ=easy, slow pace, +2=2 miles of walking

Part II – Energy/Endurance Efficiency

Week	Sun	Mon	Tue	Wed	Thu	Fri	Sat	Weekly Miles
19	4	Rest	CT	Rest	Rest	4	Rest	8
20	4 int	Rest	CT	Rest	Rest	4 EZ	Rest	12
21	11/12	Rest	2 EZ	Rest	Rest	4 EZ	Rest	17/18
22	4	Rest	CT	Rest	Rest	4	Rest	8
23	6 int	Rest	CT	4	Rest	4 EZ	Rest	14
24	6 EZ	Rest	CT	4	Rest	4 EZ	Rest	14
25	12/14	Rest	2 EZ	Rest	Rest	4 EZ	Rest	18/20
26	6	Rest	CT	4	Rest	4	Rest	14
27	6 int	Rest	CT	4	Rest	4 EZ	Rest	14
28	13/16	Rest	2 EZ	Rest	Rest	4 EZ	Rest	19/22
29	6	Rest	CT	4	Rest	4	Rest	14
30	6 int	Rest	CT	4	Rest	4 EZ	Rest	14
31	14/18	Rest	2 EZ	Rest	Rest	4 EZ	Rest	20/24
32	6	Rest	CT	4	Rest	4	Rest	14
33	6 int	Rest	CT	4	Rest	4 EZ	Rest	14
34	6 EZ	Rest	CT	4	Rest	4 EZ	Rest	14
35	16/20+2	Rest	2 EZ	Rest	Rest	4 EZ	Rest	22/24
36	6	Rest	CT	4	Rest	6	Rest	16
37	8 int	Rest	CT	4	Rest	4 EZ	Rest	16
38	18/22+2	Rest	2 EZ	Rest	Rest	4 EZ	Rest	26/30
39	6	Rest	CT	4	Rest	4	Rest	14
40	8 EZ	Rest	CT	4	Rest	4 EZ	Rest	16
41	20/24+2	Rest	2 EZ	Rest	Rest	6 EZ	Rest	28/32
42	8 EZ	Rest	CT	4	Rest	4	Rest	16
43	8 EZ	Rest	CT	4	Rest	4	Rest	16
44	8 EZ	Rest	CT	4	Rest	6 EZ	Rest	18
45	22/26+2	Rest	2 EZ	Rest	Rest	6 EZ	Rest	30/34
46	8 EZ	Rest	2 EZ	4	Rest	4	Rest	18

47	8 EZ	Rest	2 EZ	4	Rest	2 EZ	Rest	16
48	26.2	Rest	2 EZ	Rest	Rest	Total Mileage		631/657

You may be saying right now, wow, that's a shitload of running. Exactly. If you don't want to run that much, then just do a half-marathon. The marathon is not to be taken lightly. It is the real deal, and countless people get injured, many permanently. That's the whole point of my book. If, like a typical consumerist American, you want instant results for a lot of money, get liposuction.

My schedule starts out with two weeks between long runs up until ten miles. Your long runs should start very slowly and maintain a slow pace. The purpose is not speed but endurance. Slow means slow. You should be able to have a conversation at this speed. After hitting 10 miles, I give you three or four weeks of recovery between long runs. Marathoners may scoff at my one-mile increment slow start, but keep in mind, this is for the average person who is usually overweight and has never run in proper shoes. The slow initial period is designed to allow your body to slowly adapt and recover and develop muscle memory and endurance strength. There should be no stress on your joints or ligaments. If you find yourself able to run further, feel free to run further, but try to only add one-mile increments until you hit 10 miles. You may feel stronger, but you simply have to trust your body. Your body is literally injured after a long run. Muscles are torn up, and your immune system is weaker. You should take it easy, especially if you have never run long distance before. Do not push yourself. Learn to enjoy running first, and then we will get into the 10+ mile long distance runs.

After 10 miles, your body is being pushed pretty hard, so now you should expect to get worse sores, stiffness, and injury. Guess what? That's your body telling you to take it easy. Other training schedules give you only two weeks between long runs (except the last one which is three weeks before the marathon), and they keep telling you to do high mileage and intervals, but this is exactly how I got injured! After 10 miles, you need to be super, extra careful not to push yourself too hard. The only time you are ever pushing yourself hard is the long runs, otherwise, every other workout is part of your recovery, even your speed work. The three and four week intervals also allow you to fail two or three times. If you didn't hit 14 miles, no big deal, try again next week and you'll still have two weeks to recover until your next long run. The only exception to this is the last three weeks. If you miss your final long-run target, don't worry and just recover. So long as you hit the long run target before that, you'll be fine. There are four-week recovery periods in there to allow for missed long-run targets but also to allow your body to fully recover and also give you a break from long runs.

Let us be realistic. You have different priorities in life, and throughout your training, you will move around priorities. The four-week recovery periods allow you to take care of other matters in your life you may have been neglecting. Marathoners may scoff at my long schedule, but I challenge them to test this against their one and see if their injury rate is lower and their marathon completion rate is higher.

The short 20-week schedule is used to encourage people to run marathons. Telling someone it will take a year would discourage many people who are all about short-term goals and instant gratification. A 48-week training schedule will weed out people who are not truly serious and do not want to run the rest of their lives. It also significantly reduces the pressure which adds to stress which lengthens your recovery time and makes you even more vulnerable to injury. Finally, it allows you to truly assess your marathon capabilities long before signing up for a marathon.

Finding a Marathon to Run

When searching for a marathon, the most important factor is the time they allow you to finish. I believe that the average person will finish his/her first marathon in six hours both running and walking. Make sure your first marathon gives you sufficient time to finish. The second most important factor is the course difficulty. Your first marathon should have an easy course not one that is all uphill at high altitude. Don't be fooled by marathons that are mostly downhill, because running downhill actually puts tremendous stress on your joints and may lead to early joint pain and fatigue. Ideally, pick a flat course with occasional hills.

Don't register now! Unless, you're really set on the marathon and openings are running out, you should wait until you can run 10 miles before registering. Your body will tell you if you can run a marathon or not before your 10-mile run. Also, keep in mind, you will discover new aches and pains throughout your body before the 10-mile run, but unless it is acute, sharp, incessant pain, most aches and pains will naturally go away as your body strengthens not only muscles but ligaments and tendons. Never underestimate your body's ability to adapt, but at the same time, never ignore your body when you get incessant, sharp, debilitating pain. Occasional acute, sharp pain is fine. Frequent generalized, dull pain is fine. Incessant sore muscles are fine. When I started training, I had acute, sharp knee joint pain, but it eventually went away. I also had back spasms and a back strain, and they too went away, although, in hindsight, I should have waited until I fully recovered from my back strain to continue training, however, I had already signed up for the marathon. Do as I say, not as I do.

Some marathons do not allow MP3 players or smart phones with headphones so make sure that if you really need them that the marathon allows them.

Running Gear

Wear cotton in the heat and polyester in the winter. Some people will say wear polyester in the heat, but I have a problem with this. We sweat to cool ourselves. Polyester mesh takes sweat off our skin and then makes it evaporate. We may be drier, but we're also hotter. A sweat-soaked cotton shirt, at least for me, helps me cool down. The only drawback is that it will be slightly heavier and it may cause chaffing at longer distances. In the cold, the last thing you want is a sweat-soaked shirt, so polyester mesh is perfect, although, I think the very outer layer should be a natural breathable material like a cotton hoodie not a polyester fleece jacket unless it's raining in which case it's better to have rainproof material. Even then, the rainproof jacket should have slits and/or mesh vents to allow your skin to breath. You should not wear cotton socks which trap moisture and contribute to fungus and blisters. You should wear acrylic and/or polyester socks. You should also always wear poly underwear in the winter and for long distance. I can't tell you how many times I came home from a long run in the winter with underwear filled with a pound of sweat.

You should wash your polyester mesh clothing in cold water and let them air dry. They are of course specifically designed to air dry. Obviously, you can tell how good your clothes are at evaporating moisture by how quickly they dry and even how wet they feel right out of the washer.

In the cold you definitely want headgear since a disproportionate amount of heat is lost through your head. With the sun out, I wear a golf-type visor. Hats will trap skull heat. I also use sun protection lotion for longer runs.

In cold weather, you also lose a lot of heat through your hands, so wear at least a base layer of mesh poly and I would recommend an outer layer of wool/natural fibers. The mesh poly lifts moisture away from your skin, but if you have a fleece or un-breathable poly material over that, the moisture has nowhere to go but right back into the base glove.

Time-Keeping Watch

At first, I used a basic stopwatch watch and then used my iPhone to enter the lap times. I recently bought a Casio WS220-1A Solar Runner watch that stores 120 lap/split records. Let's say I run 10 miles on a 1-mile/lap course. I hit start, after lap 1 I hit the lap button and it records the time for the first lap. The overall clock keeps going on the bottom of the screen, but now on the main screen it shows my time for the 2nd lap starting at 0:00. So every lap, I know how fast I'm going, and in the end, not only do I have the total 10-mile time, but I have the time for each lap.

Smart phone or MP3 Player

Unless you can find a group or partner to run with, I would strongly urge you to use an MP3 player or better yet a smart phone and get the Pandora app. The music both kills the boredom but also sometimes gives you a nice tempo. It especially helps when you're in pain and a great song comes along to give you a little ethereal boost. I already love trance music, but I think trance music is not only perfect for raves but endurance running.

Running Location

Ideally, you can switch around your running locations to give you variety, but I trained exclusively on a 2-mile path around a lake. It helped me get an idea of exactly how fast I was running, and I could pause every lap to go to my car and rehydrate or shed or add clothing. It is absolutely crucial that if you run a marathon on pavement that you train on pavement. You can switch around with dirt trails, but over half your training and all your long runs should be pavement to train your body to deal with the incessant pounding of a hard surface. I would also arm myself just in case you run across a rabid dog or some deranged criminal.

Training

Once you start training, you need to gradually become more focused and disciplined with everything you do. You have to gradually cut back your alcohol, partying, any behavior that adds toxins into your body and causes stress and strain.

Nutrition

You need to gradually eat more quality, whole, organic, grass-fed meat, hormone and antibiotic-free food. If you already eat quality food, you will gradually eat more quality food. If all you eat is junk, you will increase your quality food intake while proportionally decreasing your junk food intake. You definitely need more quality protein not only for more energy but also to rebuild broken muscle tissue and build up your ligaments and tendons. You definitely want to increase intake of fresh fruits and vegetables to ensure that you are getting all your daily recommended doses of vitamins and minerals in addition to fiber to help you digest all your proteins. At the very least, you should take supplemental vitamins. Although, they are inferior to natural food, they are better than nothing. I take a multi-vitamin, B-12, and Zinc. I also take protein shakes after long runs and whenever I skip meat for a day. I honestly don't believe it's healthy to eat meat daily. Digesting flesh takes up a lot of your immune system that you will need to fight off colds or flu's especially when you train harder and become more stressed. So long as you are not eating junk food, you should lose fat. You may not necessarily lose weight if the muscle you gain is matched by the fat you lose. You will also lose fat around your organs, so even if you cannot see the fat diminish around your waist or thighs, you could be losing all the fat around your organs.

As you add mileage, your body will start to crave food more, any kind of food. Fight the temptation to eat junk food and stick to quality food. The added fat and toxins in junk food will only delay recuperation and add unnecessary weight for the marathon.

Always eat 100 calories before any long run to give you basic energy. For long runs, you should carb load the day before at midday. Carb loading does not mean eat until you want to throw up. It simply means two portions of carbs. I do not recommend sleeping on a full stomach, because it might wake you up when sugars are released and it robs your body of energy to digest all the food. I would also avoid meat just in case it's bad and gives you indigestion which not only flushes your proteins but also your carbs. Indigestion and diarrhea also dehydrates you. Instead, drink a protein shake the day before your long run. There are countless stories of marathon runners eating bad meat the day before and cramping or getting diarrhea the next morning. Better yet, bring your own meal for the day before so you know it will be safe. There's a story of Greg LeMond racing in the Tour de France. He ate Mexican food flown in for him and then had a horrible case of diarrhea the next day. Since he couldn't pull over and relieve himself, he had to take his teammate's cap and relieve himself into it while riding his bicycle. His teammate told him to keep the cap.

I would also carb load with slow carbs. The only time you should ever eat fast carbs is right before, during, and after a long run. Otherwise, you should only be eating slow carbs: vegetables, beans, nuts, chickpeas, whole grain, oats, and brown/wild rice. (I wouldn't eat too many beans, broccoli, or cabbage the day before the race since it will cause bloating and gas.)

Know How Much to Push Yourself

There is no doubt that people simply never push themselves enough. The majority of Americans are unhealthy and overweight. It is quite obvious that they do not exercise, because the slightest amount of physical discomfort is unbearable for them. I would guess that 1 in 10 Americans cannot push past the discomfort ceiling and do not exercise on a regular basis. 1 in 100 cannot push past the pain ceiling and plateau, but with natural aging, that plateau is actually a gradual incline down to death.

I've had people tell me that back pain is eternally recurring and every human only gets so many miles on their joints before they fail. This is all self-defeating nonsense. The human body was not invented when you were born. It is the result of not only 200K years of human evolution but 50 million years of primate evolution, 200 million years of mammal evolution, 500 million years of fish evolution, and 3.6 billion years of cellular evolution. You would think in that time period we would learn a thing or two about pushing our bodies to the limit and going beyond. There is this silly myth that it is the human conscious mind that allows humans to push themselves beyond their natural limits and achieve unnatural levels of physical performance. Hogwash. By all standards and measures, we are far from the strongest animal or have the greatest endurance. As you push yourself to the limit, you'll notice that your conscious mind leaves you and what you are left with is pure animal drive. In fact, it is the conscious mind that often messes you up by pushing you when you are injured or stopping you when you are just tired and can actually go further. Great athletes often say that when they think too much, they choke. More people would enjoy exercising if they just learned to shut off their conscious minds and be in the moment.

It is essential that you learn to push yourself past discomfort and then past dull pain, fatigue, exhaustion, and self-doubt. However, if you feel sharp, acute pain and it starts to zing or zap like an electric shock, simply stop. Never be afraid to throw away a planned day of training. I had back spasms and made the mistake of taking a muscle relaxant and then running two miles. My back only got worse. One step forward, two steps back. If I had just skipped that day of training, I would have taken one step back but two steps forward later.

Your body and mind will play games with you as you start pushing yourself. They act like children. When they encounter something uncomfortable, they will scream and throw a tantrum. If you stop and give in to them, you are only spoiling them. You must learn to ignore the screaming and the tantrum and forge ahead. It is not their discipline that is in question but yours; it is not their pain threshold in question but yours. Most people do not realize that if you push yourself past discomfort, your body and mind actually quiet down.

As you discover pain, your body and mind will act up again. They will scream and throw another tantrum. This is when most people stop. You have the majority of Americans who will quit after discomfort and become unhealthy and overweight. Then you have a minority that will exercise, but only until they feel pain, so they simply plateau. They will jog only two miles a week until they get old, and then as their body deteriorates, they will reduce that to one mile then a walk then nothing and die. Only a very small percentage of people will push on beyond the pain. Only a very small percentage will then discover a whole new world beyond pain. It is a world of endorphins and natural body chemicals that reduces pain and induces euphoria. Of course, many people get there artificially, but if you get there naturally, you are building up your body and mind not destroying it. There are no shortcuts in life. We don't get naturally high for nothing. I'm sure throughout our evolution, many humans got naturally high for nothing, but they probably never did much work and not only became weak but never found a mate with which to reproduce. Perhaps one day, we will have robots do everything for us and reproduction will not be necessary, then we can get artificially high all day long, but until that day comes, it is healthier for you to get high through pain and build your muscles up.

One day, for whatever reason, I decided to push myself beyond the pain and run 10 miles for the first time in my life for the heck of it. The pain was unimaginable. I had never suffered that much pain for as long as I can remember. Perhaps bad food poisoning was worse, a bad hangover was worse, or bad food poisoning coupled with a hangover. However, it was almost an addictive pain. I have yet to purposefully eat bad seafood and binge drink to recreate the agonizing pain of vomiting and diarrhea all night long. After about a week, I had forgotten about how awful the running pain was, and I actually craved the feeling. What I was actually craving were the endorphins that were released to counter the pain. Of course, it is tricky, because when you are training for a marathon, you only want to push yourself past the pain threshold on long runs. Otherwise, if your body is in pain, you should listen and scale back the training. For instance, if you have terrific acute, sharp pain, don't run. If you feel under the weather and simply fatigued, push yourself to run at least two miles and see if you feel better. However, for your long run, if you feel under the weather and fatigue, go as long as you can to target. It never ceases to amaze me how I'll start off with a stiff back or simply feeling lethargic or sick, and after six or eight miles, I feel fine. Believe it or not, sometimes your body will feign injury to get out of training. In the military, this happens to recruits all the time. They get back strains, ankle sprains, colds anc they actually do believe they are ill, but they don't realize that in most cases their body is playing tricks on them. This is often why drill sergeants ignore recruits complaining of illness up until the point where the recruit actually throws up or almost passes out.

Unfortunately, some recruits really are sick as portrayed in the move *A Few Good Men* where some Marine was truly sick and was punished for lagging behind. It's a difficult line to call. Unfortunately, people often confuse acute and general pain. General muscle fatigue and exhaustion hurts everywhere not any specific, localized point. You can get past general pain, but when you feel specific, pinpoint pain, especially muscle spasms, you should stop. Even more important, you should take a break and rest and only return to training when the acute pain is indecipherable. Too many people return to training too early and think the mild, acute pain will eventually go away, but it is like stretching a rubber band that has been cut midway through. Eventually, it will break. If possible, switch to an exercise that does not involve the painful area. For example, if you get a mild ankle sprain, ride a bicycle or elliptical. Never take painkillers before training!

Posture

Nobody likes being told to sit up straight, roll their shoulders back, stick out their chest, and lift their head up. But believe it or not, there was good reason old people told you to do this. This odd, pretentious, stuck-up posture is actually the best possible posture for your back. If you have ever suffered incessant back pain or soreness, you know that sitting like this is more comfortable and causes less pain. Although, you look like someone rammed a rod up your butt, you really are minimizing stress and strain on your back. I used to tweak my back whenever I sneezed, and I learned that if I arch my back first, I never tweak my back sneezing. Likewise, when you run, you want to minimize stress and strain on your back, so just like when you are sitting, your back should be straight, shoulders back, chest out, head up. Do not fall forward into your next step except when you are going up a hill. Even then, if you saw yourself from the side, your spine would be perpendicular to the horizon. As you start to tire, it is only natural to lower your heavy and huge head; however, you are only stretching your back muscles making them more susceptible to stress and strain. If you can see your feet, either you are kicking your feet far too forward or your head is down. You should never be able to see your feet. Occasionally, however, you do want to check on your feet. Make sure they are pointed straight ahead and not to the sides or inward.

While you often see professional marathoners bouncing all over the place, for them, a marathon is a race. They're going for speed. If you were to only race two-miles, you would also be bouncing all over. However, if you told the professional marathon runner to run 100 miles, he would definitely have a less bouncy, shorter stride. For endurance running, you want to shorten and lower your stride, almost to the point of shuffling. By doing this, you conserve energy as well as lessen joint pain by reducing impact on your feet.

As you run, your body will at first loosen up but then later tighten up. Try to loosen your shoulders up by occasionally pulling them up to your ears and then shake your arms out.

Drugs

Let's start with illegal, recreational drugs. I'm not saying all drugs are bad. Some drugs are like birthday cake. It is okay to do it once a year. However, habitual drug use causes your body to rely on the drug and not your natural drug manufacturing ability. Over time, your body forgets how to make its own drugs. Most people think our natural endorphins kick in only when facing excruciating, relentless pain, but what they fail to realize is that we get small bumps for low-level, sustained pain. And people often forget that this includes boredom. Boredom is painful. Evolution has created the pain to push us to act and attempt to achieve a goal. If boredom were neutral or pleasureful, we would all be sitting at home doing nothing all day. However, if we are trapped and cannot escape the boredom, our bodies release small bumps of endorphins and serotonin to help us cope. Drug addicts don't get these natural bumps, so it is no surprise that drug addicts find boredom unbearable and cannot stay in school, work for eight hours a day, or endure any sustained effort toward any long-term goal. Again, trust nature, trust your body.

As far as legal drugs, do not take muscle relaxants or painkillers before or while running. Trust your body. If you have muscle spasms or are in real pain, do not mask it. You should be able to feel it so that if it is unbearable, it is a sign to stop. Of course, for the actual marathon, after 20 miles, it may be worth it to take painkillers to finish the marathon and suffer greatly afterwards. Some experts say that ibuprofen is not good for you and only effective at reducing inflammation after high dosages (as much as 800 mg). If you need a painkiller, take aspirin instead. I also use Icy-Hot on my back although you might want the one without the intense scent which tends to linger. Unless, you are psychotic or seriously sick, you should also avoid your usual prescription drugs. Any artificial, physiologically altering substance you put into your body destabilizes your natural physiology and often adds toxins.

I'm telling you honestly that I took methylphenidate (AKA Ritalin) at the end of my marathon and my mile splits went down, but I am almost positive that it caused me to cramp at Mile 23 since it greatly dehydrated me. Huge doses of caffeine or any stimulant for that matter will also dehydrate you. Of course, if you're on top of Mount Everest and a half-mile from basecamp and ready to die, perhaps you would risk amphetamines over dehydration.

EPO is erythropoietin and tricks your body into creating more red blood cells which significantly improves your endurance. The only known side-effect is that with all the red blood cells in your blood weighing it down, it could cause your heart to stop. If you're an amateur runner, obviously, there is no point messing with it. Blood transfusion before a marathon? After a while, you have to be asking yourself: I'm running a marathon to prove to myself and others that I have the NATURAL ability to finish one not the technology, money, connections, and drugs to finish one. Stick to the low-tech stuff like carb gels, moderate caffeine, and moderate painkillers.

Long Run Training (AKA LSD: Long Slow Distance)

Slow the fuck down. When I ran 10 miles, I made the mistake of starting out doing intervals. I also kept up a fast pace in the beginning. Then I naturally tightened my knee joint and also bonked. Your long runs are only meant to build up your endurance so take it easy. The entire time, you should be able to carry on a conversation with someone or your imaginary friend. You should never feel like you're really pushing it until the last two miles. If you are starting to get tired, slow down. Don't maintain the same pace, maintain the same effort. If you go uphill or into a headwind, slow down. I would also slow down going downhill to avoid pounding your joints.

Put Band-Aids on your nipples to avoid nipple chaffing.

You may also get black toenails. This is no cause for alarm unless it spreads or starts to smell. It's a common result of repetitive stress between the toenail and toe which causes separation and internal bleeding. It often goes away after a few weeks.

For your long runs, it is essential that you take in 100 calories of fast carbs for every four to six miles. I think carb gels are perfect. The major limitation on short runs is your respiratory ability or fitness level (0-4 miles). The major limitation on medium runs is muscle fatigue (4-10 miles). The major limitation on long runs is depletion of fuel/energy (10+ miles). When you run out of water, your body becomes thirsty and your mouth becomes dry. It is easy to know when you are dehydrated. However, when your body runs out of energy, you don't become hungry. You simply crash and burn, what is referred to as bonking or hitting the wall. It is like someone put a 50-lb. backpack on you or took away half your oxygen. As you push on, you'll feel light-headed, disoriented, confused, sick, you may dry heave and you'll feel pain all over your body all at once. Your body is telling you to stop and collapse.

You should also drink 12 oz before your long run and at least six oz every four miles. After four miles, I would switch to a drink that includes electrolytes (salt) which is basically Gatorade, but I prefer G2 Gatorade which has much less sugar. You should then drink 12 oz after the run. You should also eat fast carbs immediately after the run to immediately restore your energy, then drink a protein drink, settle for an hour and then eat a full meal but do not overdo it. You need energy to rebuild tissue not just digest food.

For long runs, I take a small break every two miles to drink Gatorade and stretch. At 16+ miles, I take a small break every four miles to stretch. I now take carb gels every six miles, but it all depends on you, your weight, and how fast you process carbs.

For long runs, take a warm-hot shower to loosen your muscles. Never stretch cold muscles. Warm up for a hundred yards or so and then stretch. Also, 20% of a long run should be a warm up and 10% should be a warm down. In other words, if you run 10 miles, the first two miles should be extremely easy as well as the last mile. If you run 20 miles, the first four miles should be warm up and the last two should be warm down.

The name of the game with endurance running is calm. I used to be a bicycle sprinter in high school, and the name of the game was abrupt, explosive, chaotic, rage-induced madness. It is no wonder that personality types follow certain types of sport. With sprinting, it would help to build up a lot of anger, rage, and intensity before a sprint and then use the sprint to release it all. Sprinting is basically a self-induced, violent, controlled epileptic fit, panic attack orgasm. Endurance running is the complete opposite. Pent up anger and intense emotions constantly release toxins into your blood stream that undermines your recovery and tightens your muscles leading to greater stress and strain. While you are running, anger and intense emotions distract you and make you hold your breath unconsciously and puts lactic acid into your blood. As an endurance runner, you have to exercise mental endurance and patience and calm like a Zen monk. You cannot let anything bother or stress you. In this way, endurance running can be very therapeutic. It forces you to calm yourself and relax. There is immediate negative feedback when you start to panic and stress out, you immediately feel more tired and exhausted. It is no wonder that endurance fitness is better at reducing depression than drugs or therapy. It was this realization that made long distance running one of my best life experiences. Instead of stressing about not being able to finish a marathon because of my knee or back pain, I learned to simply calm down, relax, and have a little patience and faith in myself. Simply by doing this, my knee pain and back spasms disappeared, although, the back soreness lasted longer. I also learned the critical connection between patience and faith. Whenever I find myself impatient, I also realize that I have very little faith in myself or others.

I also quickly learned exactly where and when I stress out leading to back stiffness. The number one place is work. Number two is a crowded public place. Number three is heavy traffic. Every time I stressed out about the marathon, my back became stiffer while every time I simply learned to relax, it became looser. It is interesting to note that when I started running long-distance my body would fall into disarray and in that exhausted fragile state; I realized everything about modern life that caused more stress and suffering. In our normal state, the stresses of modern life are just taken for granted, but in a weakened state you really feel it physically and start to realize what it is about modern life that is truly stressful and unhealthy:

The Unhealthy Stresses of Modern Life

1. Modern work. Back in the day, we had a lot more autonomy. We worked in small teams. There were small attainable daily goals as well as long-term goals. It was more physically demanding. The leaders were those with more experience and charisma for getting the job done not a bunch of anti-social assholes who put their social lives aside to make the most money they could get their grubby hands on. Today's leaders are simply people who could do their work well and not truly lead people.

2. Sitting on your ass all day. This is unhealthy. I think about half the physical stress of work comes from simply sitting on your ass all day. And as much as you try to keep your back straight, it always tends to slouch. These days I take a lot more breaks to walk around even if I'm not thirsty I'll take a trip to the water cooler.

3. Big crowds. Animals don't like to be penned up in large crowds so why would humans? Overcrowding stresses animals so why wouldn't it stress humans? America has done a great job preparing kids for the modern world by cramming them all into gigantic high school campus warehouses which causes unnaturally high levels of stress and damage to them both psychologically and physically. People love big cities for the diversity, culture, wealth, and opportunities, but they often don't realize it all comes at the cost of the stress caused by incessant, large crowds.

4. Traffic. No animal travels continually at 65 or 75 MPH. The human has not adapted to traffic hence 40,000 Americans die each year in traffic, hence road rage. I keep telling myself that 90% of the drivers out there are worse than me, and I should calm down and forgive them, but truth is, I'm probably more in the middle and piss off as many people as piss me off. Truth is the constant dangers, the high speeds, the waiting, the continual hand-eye coordination demands all add up to big stress.

5. Excessive partying and intoxicants. Okay, so I may be unnaturally gifted in this department, but I have to believe that the first four stresses play a big part in the fifth. Perhaps back in the day, after an unsuccessful hunt or a poor crop harvest, people partied a little to unwind, but in our modern world it seems people need to unwind constantly and excessively. It seems the mind numbing characteristics of school, work and the modern life are played out in a gruesome pantomime satire while partying until you black out. Then the irony sets in when the partying itself becomes a big source of stress.

6. Traveling. Okay, traveling is wonderful but fact is, for humans, it is unnatural. We are nomadic but we don't go visiting other villages in completely other parts of the world regularly. When we travel, instinctively we worry about possible new threats, native hostility, food sources, a place to sleep, shelter. Of course, in our minds we have everything set with reservations, but our bodies become all tight and stressed in any new environment. There's a reason they call it home turf advantage.

7. Sleeping on a soft mattress and eating fast carb's and sugar or taking stimulants before bed. When I had back spasms, I tended to lie in bed quite a bit, and ironically, I'd wake up with a stiffer back than when I went to bed. Soft beds are like cushioned shoes. They are unnatural and actually hurt us. We think it may be nice to sleep on a nice, cushy bed, but this induces us to roll around more, further injuring our muscles, tendons, and ligaments. On a firm mattress, or even sleeping on the floor, your body cannot roll as much. Your body instantly feels the feedback of a hard surface and stops. Also, when we sleep, we are partially paralyzed to keep us from rolling too much or acting on our dreams, but if we take sugars or stimulants before we sleep, they can actually overrule our paralysis or simply create more exciting dreams that cause us to act them out more.

Not to be totally negative, but was there anything that helped reduce my soreness and stiffness in modern life instead of exacerbate them? I would offer the following:

- Moderate alcohol, partying and hanging out with friends

- Healthy organic eating

- Proper sleep and rest

- Distance from the office. Seriously, my back pains would miraculously disappear once I left the office.

Speed Training

Every other week, you should do speed training. This does not mean sprinting. Sprinting is the opposite of marathon running or training. This is like practicing for a ping pong game by trying to bench 400 lbs. Sprinting will simply build up muscle bulk and fast-twitch muscles which will be useless and even hinder you in a marathon. Speed training is designed to increase your cardiovascular fitness, your body's ability to take in oxygen and distribute it effectively. When you sprint, you often hold your breath and use up lactic acid for fuel. If you find yourself holding your breath, you are running too fast. Sprinting also causes huge stress on your joints as you basically strike the ground with your feet. Imagine punching the ground with your fists and the stress it would put on your wrists. Speed training is running for half-a-mile as fast as you can without losing breath. At the end, your lungs should be bursting and screaming at you. Then jog lightly until your breathing is restored to normal and go another half-mile. You should speed train for less than 50% the distance of your last long run. You should stop doing intervals 11 weeks before the marathon to avoid possible injury. With 11 weeks to go, all you need to do is sustain cardiovascular fitness and work on extending endurance and energy conservation/efficiency.

Strength Training

If you lift weights, you should lift weights up until 11 weeks to go.
However, you shouldn't do grunting, six rep, heavy lifting. If you lift
weights regularly, cut your weights in half and double your reps. You
want to build lean muscle not bulk. Also, you do not want to risk
straining or spraining anything especially with 11 weeks to go. You
definitely need to work all your muscles since you will be working all your
muscles in a marathon. I would also recommend yoga which exercises
tiny muscles you simply cannot reach with regular weights. Whenever any
muscle, no matter how small, gets fatigued and starts using lactic acid, that
lactic acid circulates through your entire body. You don't want any
muscle, no matter how small to get fatigued. Of most importance, you
should work your stomach and back muscles, your core, however, use
very light weights on your back muscles to avoid a back strain. The last
11 weeks, do not try any new type of exercise as it may result in a strain.
With 11 weeks to go, all your running muscles will be sore and fatigued
and they are more vulnerable than ever to being overstretched and
strained.

Time of Day

Run whenever it is convenient for you to run. It does not matter if it is
early morning, midday, or evening. Exercise is exercise. Also, some
people will tell you to avoid running in the midday heat, but so long as
you keep hydrated, you will adapt to running in heat just use a lot of sun
screen. Keep in mind, many long-distance runners come from all
different climate zones of the world and become champions. Nordic
skiers, arguably athletes with the greatest endurance, train in the cold
while Kenyan runners train in the heat. Also keep in mind, while

Americans have the benefit of the best technology: shoes, clothing, carb gels, Gatorade, etc., many amateur Kenyans have none of that and could easily kick your ass. You do get a small benefit from technology, but fundamentally, it is your determination and consistent motivation that matters more than anything else.

Last Long Distance Run

Your last long distance run should be run as if it was the marathon. The day before should be exactly like the day before your marathon. Get up at the exact same times, eat the exact same foods, do the exact same things. When you get to the marathon starting line, you often stand around for an hour, so stand around for a while before you train. Shorten all your breaks.

Injury

You will get injured if you push yourself too hard too soon. It's as simple as that. The hardest things to know for certain is how much to push yourself, because sometimes, you discover that you can push yourself a lot harder than you ever thought, and sometimes you discover that you cannot push yourself anywhere near as much as you thought. Keep in mind, sharp, acute pain is always bad. Stop. Incessant dull pain, soreness, and stiffness are okay. General pain and discomfort is nothing. You are pushing yourself too much if you cannot get over the same pain problem. If you have a painful knee or ankle, try keeping up fitness for a week by bicycling or another aerobic activity with minimum pressure on your knees and ankles. You are pushing yourself just right when your specific pain problem goes away after a week. It took me one month to get rid of my back spasms, so I was probably pushing myself too hard. Also keep in mind, failing to finish a marathon is a onetime defeat, a single day's disaster. That's all. All that training is not a waste, because after you recover, not only will you have all your experience, but you will not go back to Week 1. When you are fully recovered, you will discover that you can probably cut the 48-week training session in half for your next marathon attempt. Also, your next marathon attempt, you are more likely to jog the entire way. Think of it this way. Some people finish two marathons. The first they jog and walk, and the second they jog all the way. You only finish one marathon, but you jogged the entire way. While you may hate the fact that you'll have to do all those long 12+ mile runs again, it's also quite possible that you'll realize that you enjoy long-distance running. People who finish their first marathon on their first try often will never run another marathon, but after training for two marathons, it is more likely that you'll run a third marathon and make long-distance running a lifestyle. Lastly, I have met people who pushed themselves too hard in any athletic endeavor and have life-long injuries. It just isn't worth it.

The Gift of Pain and Fear

Wouldn't it be great not to feel pain? You might become a super-athlete capable of extraordinary feats of human strength and endurance. You would be fearless. You would live without worries or heartburn. Wouldn't you be truly free and liberated? Don't you often wonder whether the only difference between you and Olympians and world champions is that somehow, they have a diminished sense of pain? There actually are people who have a significantly diminished ability to sense pain. Far from being super-athletes, they are all crippled for life. They poke their eyeballs until they are blind, they walk on broken legs, they tear skin off their body, they chew into their tongues, they twist their fingers back and break them. Lack of pain is one of the worst afflictions you could suffer. Pain is a gift, yet we are so prone to ignore it and over-medicate it. The slightest discomfort and we succumb to the urge of eating garbage, abusing drugs, alcohol, abusing stimulants at the slightest sense of fatigue and abusing sedatives at the slightest sense of anxiety. Instead of heeding the warning signs of pain that we may be working too hard, exercising too hard, not sleeping long enough, not recovering long enough, partying too hard, hanging around hurtful people, being lonely, etc., we ignore the pain and try to erase it artificially. Like people genetically incapable of feeling pain, we too are becoming crippled by our inability to honestly feel pain.

If you learn one thing training for a marathon, it will be pain. But if you make the most of it, you will not ignore or cloak the pain with drugs. You will feel it, respect it, endure it, and respond to it. Injury often occurs when you ignore or cloak pain. And people ignore and cloak pain, because they have a fear of pain. However, what we all forget are two things. When we suffer pain, our bodies provide us with natural painkillers: endorphins. And if we respond to the pain by backing off and resting, the pain goes away. Like most people, I would hate to not finish my first marathon and go through hell training for another one, but fact is, if I avoid injury this time around, I will be better prepared to train for another one, and while there will be another tremendous round of pain, there will also be another round of natural painkillers, and if I recover fully, I'll simply be stronger for the next marathon. Don't let pain and fear get the better of you. When humans project into the future, they suffer from the inability to appreciate the law of diminishing returns. If you imagined eating a gigantic buffet, you would imagine relishing every single morsel equally, but in reality, your appreciation of each bite diminishes with time. Your body must do this to prevent you from overeating or eating the same nutrient and ignoring other nutrients. Your body craves variety. Likewise, when we imagine confronting a spouse, boss, or getting in a fight, we imagine recoiling from every stinging insult or blow. In reality, the pain also diminishes so that you can overcome and grow strong. Never overestimate pleasure or pain.

If anything, my hypothesis is that super athletes are not just gifted with natural endurance and strength but also a heightened sense of pain. What? Yes, a heightened sense of pain. This prevents them from over-training when they're injured and creating career-ending injuries. This also makes their body more likely to release endorphins quicker and in larger quantities thereby getting them hooked quicker and more intensely. A heightened sense of pain is also related to hypersensitivity in general, and I believe super athletes are not only hypersensitive to pain and endorphins, but they are also hypersensitive to the rewards of success: the accolades, attention, fame, glory, competition, and subtle tactics and techniques of the game. Also, being hypersensitive to criticism, failure, abuse, and disappointment, they are driven even more to succeed.

Last Three Weeks

You are done building up anything. You should not be building up anything anymore. You should simply be maintaining now and doing everything easy. Your body is busy at work repairing everything and needs as much rest and fuel. You will not lose any fitness so long as you keep running and exercising lightly and regularly. The last three weeks, you should be on perfect behavior. Tell all your friends and family that you have three, two, one week to go and you can't go out to that party or music festival or water park or whatever. This is when you should be the most selfish. This is your biggest test. Don't throw one of those *One Flew over the Cuckoo Nest* deals if you know what I'm talking about. You've invested far too much to blow it now. Keep stress to a minimum, keep novelties to a minimum, and eat only the best food around. Don't try any new restaurants or foods that may give you food poisoning depriving your body of a few days of essential nutrients and vitamins to rehabilitate your body. No more binge drinking and 3 AM partying. No more recreational drugs except pot which is more medicinal than recreational. No more crowds or kids where you can get some cold or even worse, the flu. If training up to now was a test in pushing yourself forward, now is the test for restraining yourself back. Get to sleep early each night. Pretend you are the biggest goodie-two-shoe in the universe. You may start to get cabin fever, but this boredom and restlessness is good and will build up energy reserves for the marathon. From personal experience I can tell you that eating more healthy proteins speeds recovery and drinking all night leaves me sore and stiff the next morning.

Week Prior

This is probably the most important week of all as well as the most stressful. It is critically important to reduce stress and keep all the negative influences out of your life. It may even help you to take a couple days off work right before the marathon weekend. I would also suggest avoiding any kind of food that may get you sick like seafood or cheap Chinese food. I speak from experience. You need all the nutrients, hydration, and rest you can get to heal everything that has been hurt. Right about now, people are thinking that they must finish the marathon with all the training, money, and pain, but keep in mind the journey is more important than the destination. You learned a lot about yourself, you pushed yourself to the limit, you survived, and even if you do not finish, you are more prepared than ever to finish next time and you will not be starting from scratch next time. Do not pressure yourself to complete the marathon. Keep in mind, the goal is to finish without sustaining a lifelong injury. Present mind impacts future performance. We do not know the future. Whatever you think of religion, faith, or science, the fact is, we do not know the future. The larger the stake, the greater the worry and stress. So if you adopt a philosophy that increases that stress, you are negatively impacting future performance. If you adopt a philosophy that decreases the stress, you are positively impacting future performance. Cockiness negatively impacts future performance, because it tricks you into resting too much and not keeping up your fitness. But now is the time to truly believe in yourself, in some greater power, in some unseen force to give you the power and will to finish that marathon. You may scoff at the lack of scientific evidence, previous injuries and failures, but keep in mind, present mind impacts future performance. It does not matter one iota if after the marathon you are proven right or wrong. That is immaterial now. Right now, you simply must bring yourself to believe in yourself right or wrong. By doing this, you are positively impacting future performance. You were meant to finish the marathon. There is no coincidence that you picked that marathon, the timing of your decision to run, the circumstances that led you to start long distance running, etc, etc, etc. Believe it was meant to be!

You may also worry that everyone will think you are a failure or quitter if you do not finish, but ask yourself, have they finished a marathon? They have no idea what it takes, and more likely, they will understand if you did not finish and will not be disappointed in you. Only bad friends will think you failed. A good friend will be proud you tried and their esteem of you will increase.

The boredom of easy and light training may also encourage you to eat more, but try to minimize fast carbs and fats that will only add weight. Eat protein, fruits, vegetables, and complex carbs. I would not eat meat three days before the marathon to protect your immune system and rather take protein shakes and vegetable protein. They even make protein shakes from brown rice. I would also significantly reduce or altogether eliminate alcohol which is often high in fast carbs and sugars and the depressant effect of alcohol in conjunction with social settings will make you vulnerable to catching colds or the flu. However, if you are a regular or excessive drinker, going cold turkey may also have temporary negative impacts on your health.

Pre-Marathon

If you are traveling to another city, ideally, you should arrive at least two days before the marathon. The day before the marathon should be no stress. Sleeping two nights in the marathon city will also acclimatize you to the altitude, weather, humidity, etc. By sleeping two nights before the marathon in a strange bed, you are more likely to sleep better the night before the marathon as well. Often you have to pick up your bib the day before the marathon, so you really do not want to risk missing a flight and then arriving late and missing the registration window. Traveling also is stressful which will tighten your muscles and put unnecessary stress toxins in your body. It may feel like a waste of money to visit a new city and not go out, but your priority is the marathon not sight-seeing. The name of the game is minimizing stress to the point of utter boredom. Minimizing stress also means planning, planning, planning. Study the map of your hotel location and marathon location. If you can, walk around the marathon start location to familiarize yourself with it. Don't pack the night before but a couple days earlier. You're bound to always forget something. Make a packing list. Carry all your essential running gear in your carryon. Carry an extra pair of shoe laces.

The Day Before

You should wake up exactly at the same time as the morning of the marathon. Do not be tempted to go out sightseeing. You should try to avoid any walking or standing of any kind. Read a book, magazine, go to a movie theater, or just sit in bed all day. While the boredom might be unbearable, you are building up both your energy and restlessness for the marathon. You want to be impatient for the marathon to start and not fear it. At midday eat a double dose of slow carbs. Try to avoid taking naps during the day which may keep you awake at night. Walk around a little to look for fruits and vegetables you can eat for dinner and in the morning. If necessary take sleeping pills so you can sleep all night. Just in case, I would set your watch alarm, your hotel alarm clock, and bring your own battery-operated alarm clock or put a fresh battery in your electric alarm clock. One alcoholic beverage the day before is fine as it will also help relax your nerves but avoid it in the evening. The sugar may wake you up at night. Don't hang out at the marathon registration or expo. You are surrounded by a huge crowd of people who have pushed themselves to the limit, and I guarantee you some of them are sick. Don't eat any of those free samples, because you never know what is in them and how you will react to them. Take them to try later or give them to your friends who supported you.

Marathon

Take a warm-hot shower. If you feel stiff, jog lightly in place to loosen your muscles. Try to get to the marathon early in case there is traffic or you get lost. Do as much as you can to relax and stay calm. One great way is to simply talk to other runners which will make the time fly faster. Standing there all by yourself will only make you nervous. Try to be calm, listen to music, but don't be stoic and anti-social. Keep loose. You see athletes right before a big event all alone, pacing, listening to music, trying to concentrate, but I'm certain that they're doing it wrong. You need to be chatting with friends and acting like it's a day like every other. The key is to be distracted and loose not overly focused and tense. Chilling with friends is the best way to stay loose and relaxed.

Everyone starts out too fast. All the crowds, energy, adrenaline make you go out fast just to get rid of all the pent up nervous energy. Slow the fuck down and pace yourself. Let the idiots and novices pass you by. If you run a marathon correctly, everyone passes you in the beginning and you will pass everyone at the end. Look around and enjoy the scenery and crowds. Smile and relax. And slow the fuck down. You cannot possibly go too slow the first two miles. If you feel you are going too slow, you're probably going just about right on target.

Should you take any artificial drugs? While caffeine is fine, I would wait until the last quarter of the marathon. You will have enough energy in the morning with all your excitement and anticipation. If anything, some people may want to take a very small dosage of anti-anxiety medication if they usually use it. If you are feeling good, you don't need anything, but with eight miles to go, if you need help, you can certainly use caffeine, painkillers, ibuprofen, etc. I made the mistake of taking 10 mg of methylphenidate (generic Ritalin) with several miles to the end. I already had taken a lot of ibuprofen for my sore ankle. At Mile 23 my left knee tendon cramped. I am pretty sure the methylphenidate dehydrated me and greatly contributed to the cramp if not caused it. 10 mg of Ritalin may not dehydrate you when you're sitting in school or at the office, but trust me, when you're running a marathon already sucking up liters of water, 10 mg will dehydrate you like a half gram of meth. So simple advice is to avoid stimulants unless you absolutely need it, and you're within a mile of the finish. I took the stimulant, because I had read a book about someone climbing Mt. Everest and they carry two emergency stimulants in case they bonk and they're near camp. Keep in mind, I was really only planning on using it in an emergency, but in my dazed and exhausted state, I wound up taking every pill of everything I brought.

I walked for a little, but then I saw this guy pass me, and he was doing this mini-jog, so I copied him and realized it was possible to do a mini-jog with my cramp so long as I didn't fully extend my left leg. It looked odd, and I always said I'd finish the marathon with my dignity, but after 23 miles, you truly don't care. I didn't want to walk the rest of the way, so I did my dopey-jog the rest of the way to the finish line. I was averaging 11 and half minutes a mile before the cramp and then about 16 minutes a mile after. I didn't hit my goal of a sub-5 hour marathon, but I thought to myself, if I had cramped at Mile 20, I would have been lucky to do sub-6 hours and if I had cramped at Mile 16, I might not have even finished. So in hindsight, I was lucky and fortunate.

After several miles, at every mile post I stopped to quickly stretch my legs for a few seconds, but I think after 20 miles, I would suggest not stopping. At this point, your legs are stiff no matter how much you stretch them, and if you stop, as I did right before cramping, you could cramp up. I would also suggest drinking three or four cups at each aid station if they are about two miles apart. The cups are often only half full, and after only taking two cups for the first half of the marathon, I realized I wasn't really drinking enough. After the marathon, I pee'd dark yellow, so I knew I was dehydrated.

All the way, I kept shaking out my arms and shoulders and tried to stay relaxed which is key. A third of the way to go, a lot of people lined the course with signs, and reading the humorous signs and chuckling to myself kept my attitude light and loose. It was only when I cramped that I grimaced and started cussing and ignored all the people cheering me and their signs. I'm also pretty sure I was in and out of consciousness the last three miles. I don't even recall much of the marathon to be honest. Perhaps that happens to a lot of people.

I would also suggest that you thank all the volunteers who give you drinks no matter how tired or in pain you are in. Without them, you wouldn't even be able to run.

Finally, when my friend told me that her husband's nuts chafed when he ran long distance, I laughed. I put Band-Aids on my nipples, but I didn't touch my balls. Well, I don't know how the hell it happens, but yes, the back of your scrotum chafes, so yes, put some Vaseline on the backside of your nutsack. The oddest thing I saw were women with their hands out offering a dollop of Vaseline. Who does that? Only in a marathon. Ever seen a woman standing on a street corner offering a free dollop of Vaseline?

Post-Marathon

If you couldn't finish, life goes on. Don't beat yourself up. The biggest part of a marathon is the training not the race. You learned more in training than you ever will during a marathon. You may not think you'll ever try to finish a marathon ever again, but give it a year and see how you feel after a year.

If you finished, you should grab some quick fast carbs, protein, and rest and then have a meal. If you want to go out and party and get drunk, go for it, but keep in mind, you're more likely to pass out and get sick since your body will be in a state of complete disorder and shock. Actually, I would just recommend light partying and then save it for the evening after and when you return home to celebrate with all your friends and family.

I went out the evening of the marathon, and in hindsight, I think I was in a weird funky, hazed, stoned state. I had three alcoholic beverages and was in a very bad mood.

The next day I went out and drank nine alcoholic beverages and passed out. It's not uncommon of me to drink nine drinks and be fine, but I definitely think I overestimated myself. After running 26.2 miles, your body is in severe disrepair, inflammation, and shock, and your immune system will be severely lowered. I wound up catching a small cold. Your mind will think your body is sore but fine, but your body is a wreck, and you should really take it easy. Take it super easy the evening of the marathon, take it easy the next day, and try not to overexert yourself the rest of the week. It will take you at least a week for your body to get back to normal. In fact, if you're lucky, get a couple days off work right after the marathon.

During the marathon, you'll suffer Marathon Memory Deficiency (MMD). I swear, I cannot remember huge chunks of the marathon, especially the ending, and I talked with other marathon finishers, and they experienced the same thing. All your energy is expended in your legs, so your frontal lobes and memory parts get a lot fewer resources to function properly.

Right after the marathon you will suffer the Post-Marathon Fog (PMF). You will feel perfectly fine and normal, but certain things just won't make sense or you'll look back on something and find it a bit off how you reacted. You'll walk around acting a bit stoned and dreamy for a bit.

A few days following the marathon, you'll get Post-Marathon Depression (PMD). Things will seem grey and dull. Life will seem boring. You'll find your grand marathon accomplishment one huge anti-climax, but what is happening is that your mind is getting your body to rest. If you felt great, you might go out and party and travel or exert yourself and not allow yourself to recover. PMD is designed to get you to lie around all depressed and devalue everything in life so you get the critical rest you need to replenish and repair your body. Don't counter-act PMD with anti-depressants, stimulants, caffeine, or therapy. Just rest and chill out. Once your body replenishes all the depleted stores of sugar, vitamins, and minerals and repairs all the damaged tissues, you will be re-energized, strong as ever. It took me about a week to get over PMD, and then the world was clear and normal again as if a fog had lifted.

You also will probably get Post-Marathon Munchies (PMM). You've basically exhausted your body's entire supply of nutrients, vitamins, and minerals. Your body will crave everything in huge quantities, but keep in mind, if you feed your body quality, natural foods it will crave less than if you just eat junk food. If you eat junk food, your body will just want larger quantities of junk food to make up for the lower percentage of nutrients.

I told everyone I would only run one marathon, but even a few days after the marathon, I was tempted to run another next year. Marathons are like anything that involves some form of intense pain like tattoos, weightlifting, even binge drinking with hangovers. While some people are immediately turned off by pain, some people like myself, get addicted to the endorphins. I don't believe it when people say they are addicted to pain. This makes no sense. It is like saying you hate pleasure. People are addicted to the endorphins your body releases when you suffer pain. This whole book tells people not to run marathons. They are unhealthy. I would also tell people not to binge drink or drink excessively either. I may run another marathon, and of course, I will probably binge drink, but if you want to be healthy, do as I say not as I do. That also points out another danger of marathons. You can become addicted to them, spend lots of money, gets lots of injuries, and wind up crippled for life.

Summary of Why You Should Not Run a Marathon

- Most all people have grown up wearing shoes that have significantly realigned and disfigured our natural, healthy stride. It has also deformed our feet. Expecting us to run a marathon is like expecting a Chinese woman with bound feet to run a mile without self-injury. We first need to slowly transition into minimalist shoes or barefoot running, and this often takes years to do so safely.

- The average American is overweight. The additional weight they bring to running adds significant stress to their joints, muscles, tendons, and ligaments significantly increasing the risk of injury.

- Many Americans are also more muscular than our Paleolithic ancestors, and muscles add extra weight which in turn adds extra stress to our joints. Even in my 5 hour corral, I don't recall seeing a big, muscle dude.

- Paleothic folks ran everywhere all their lives. Taking a sedentary, overweight creature and making it run a marathon is like taking a dolphin and teaching it how to fly.

- Most marathons have time limits that encourage participants to run hard the entire time without sufficient breaks. Running 26.2 miles without rest significantly increases the risk of injury.

- Most marathons cover only one type of terrain the entire length which causes more repetitive stress to the body increasing the risk of injury.

- Most marathons do not give people full or partial refunds if they do not participate. Many injured runners force themselves to participate in marathons to avoid the financial hit leading to greater and more lasting injuries.

- Reducing body weight to avoid injury in a marathon not only means slimming down but losing muscle mass which makes you look like a scrawny dork.

- The human head is proportionally heavier than most all other animals so perhaps people who run marathons fast with no injury have really light brain mass.

- Finally, not only can you get black toes, but one of your frickin' toenails can become completely detached from your toe, and in my case, I simply cut it out. It could take a year to completely grow back, and I hear it never becomes the pretty thing it used to be.

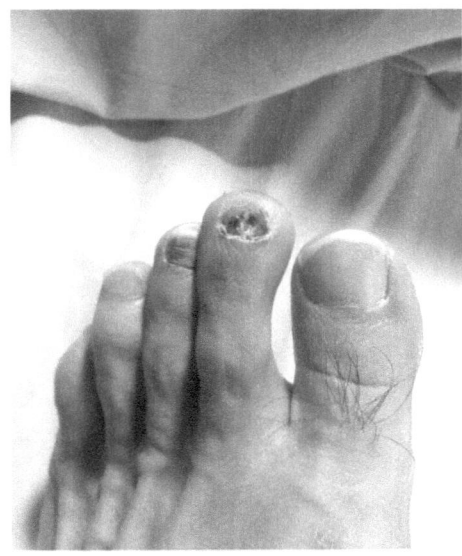

Benefits of Long-Slow-Distance (LSD) Running

Don't get me wrong. I am an opponent of the ultra-long-distance, single-terrain, non-stop marathon and not long-slow-distance running (LSD) in general. In fact, I have become an avid LSD runner. Of course, "long-distance" is all relative and true long-distance runners would consider me a middle-slow-distance runner. For my purposes, I will define long-distance as 10+ miles. Ultra-long-distance would be over 20 miles. I also happen to enjoy sprinting and my speed intervals, however, I now also enjoy long, slow, steady jogging to the point of bonking. For some people, they never get injured and might think that this book is a call for mediocrity. Some people are naturally talented runners for whatever reason. They may be genetically born with more red blood cells, absorb more calcium, have stronger ligaments, have more slow-twitch muscle fibers, have less dense and lighter bones, whatever. How many Samoan marathon runners are there? However, fact is, there are much fewer of them than people who get injured. As far as I'm concerned, more people run half-marathons, enjoy half-marathons, get injured less, and keep running, so why not promote half-marathons and leave marathons to the true athletes who can commit the time and energy to it and not the casual, average citizen?

Here are some of the benefits you can get from long-slow-distance running:

- LSD is more likely to give you a runner's high, an endorphin rush that is addictive and will more likely keep you motivated to keep fit than short-distance running.

- Running is more effective at combatting depression than therapy or drugs.

- LSD encourages you to be healthy when you are not running, because if you are not healthy outside of running, you are less likely to be able to do LSD. LSD encourages you to drink less alcohol, party fewer hours, stop partying earlier, do less recreational drugs, eat better and more natural food, be less angry and impatient, stress less, drive more safely, and be more positive at work and in your relationships.

- LSD encourages you to believe in yourself and your body's natural abilities to heal and grow. LSD has improved my faith in myself.

- LSD encourages you to be more positive and optimistic in life, to believe in positive outcomes, people, and intentions. Negativity tends to tighten your body up and slow healing and worsen physical injuries. In other words, negativity is a self-fulfilling prophecy for losers.

- LSD gives you minor injuries that make you stronger in the long run. On the other hand, marathons give you major injuries that make you weaker in the long run.

- LSD trains you to be calm, in control, patient, persevering, positive, forgiving, and willful. We tend to look for agency in life, something that caused something, and we often go external, blaming external agents for bad outcomes. LSD trains you to go internal and look for the only one agent in your life, your will.

- LSD trains you to be more in tune with your body and mind. Hey there body, didn't know you were there. Hey there mind, how you feeling today? Positive. Cool beans. LSD is like a matchmaking service introducing you to yourself. At first, you think you're ugly and prone to injury and painful to behold, but after a while, you grow on yourself and adore the cute ways you overcome hardship.

- LSD trains you to be the leader and master of your body and mind and not the follower.

- LSD trains you to succeed in the long, slow distance run called life.

- LSD spills over to any endurance work you do whether school or work. It teaches you not to panic when you encounter a big obstacle or harsh criticism and not to fear fear itself but to know that you have the hidden, untapped power within you to overcome and naturally diminish the future pain. Remember, we have diminishing returns on pleasure but also diminishing returns on pain.

- Your goal in life should be aligned with living a better, more fulfilling, more meaningful life where you contribute more to the lives of others. Therefore, LSD should be one of the activities in your life. A marathon is just a stupid, random number of miles, self-indulgent, and completing a marathon is meaningless especially if it winds up stopping you from enjoying LSD.